# HCG-DIET; WHAT DR. SIMEONS REALLY SAID

## BACK TO THE ROOTS OF HCG DIET

DAN HILD

# Contents


1. Obesity – A Disorder     1

2. Glandular Theories On Obesity     5

3. The Causes Of Obesity     7

4. Signs And Symptoms     11

5. Treating Obesity     14

6. The Gonadotrophins     17

7. Obesity Complicating Disorders     22

8. The Technique     26

9. Conclusion     41

# CHAPTER ONE

# Obesity – A Disorder

Obesity, which is thought to be a result of excessive eating and lack of physical activity, is actually a disorder of the functioning of our body. According to this aspect, it is made clear that even if a person overeats and does not have this disease, will never get fat. Hence, it is easy to understand that obesity is more like to be a disorder, than a result of habits or self-control.

According to severity, it can be divided as mild, moderate and severe. The severe form will accumulate fat rapidly while the mild form will take a long time to show an increment of weight.

This disorder affects both genders and all ages. It may have a genetic factor as well. Among them a secondary involvement of endocrine glands such as pituitary, thyroid, adrenals and sex glands plays a great role too.

According to these reasoning and facts, it is clear that obesity should be treated as a disease. The treatment should be effective in both sexes and all ages. Also, this disorder, once corrected should allow the patient to eat any food, normally, without regaining lost weight. If this goal is approachable, then we can say that we are able to cure obesity as a disease.

In the near history obesity was something which was being praised. People though that it was a sign of high status and prosperity of a man. But in early history obesity was non-existent among humans, as still in most of the wild animals. But, with the development of the world and civilization of human beings, obesity has slowly moved in to the race of human beings. Even today we can see that there is a trend, accepting obesity as an asset and a sexual selection.

Regular Meals

The civilization of human beings introduced meals into the human life style in the early Neolithic times. But before, people ate only when they were hungry and what they ate were unrefined, row and healthy.

The human gastro-intestinal tract is structured like of an ape, rat or pig which allows continuous intake of small amounts of food. But with the theory of 'meals', we pour large amount of food suddenly to our gastro-intestinal tract. Moreover, these regular meals allowed a man to eat more than he needed, just to keep him full until next meal and this surplus had to be stored in the body which we call as fat or obesity.

Three kinds of fat

There are three kinds of fats in our body. First is the structural fat, which structurally help the organs to stay in its correct place and they provide support and absorption of shocks.

The second type is the normal reserve of fuel, which supply enough energy when the energy need goes high and the intake becomes less. Fat has the highest caloric value when compared to carbohydrates and proteins. Hence, the body can produce more energy by burning fats. This is why fat has become the most economic store of fuel in a human body.

The third type of fat is the fat, which accumulate in a body of an obese person. This fat is abnormal and is also a reserve of fuel, but these fats do not supply energy in an emergency. They can be only used in a chronic fuel insufficiency of the body.

That is why an obese person will lose his normal fats first when he starves himself, then, when these fat reserves get insufficient the body uses structural facts and it is only at the end the abnormal fats are being used. This is the reason why the obese patients' complaint, that they don't lose weight, or they lose fats at the beginning of their weight loss diet. They will get exhausted and some would have even stopped dieting before they reach the stage of losing abnormal fats at last.

These obese people feel tired, their faces become haggard, but their belly, hips, thighs and arms show to be a little leaner than earlier. The wrinkles appear and give an older look. This really exhausts people and can be one of the worst experiences of life.

Obese – being blamed

Another thing which obese people have to bear is the injustice of being accused of so many things such as greed, cheating and sexual selections. Once they determine to give up overcoming obesity, they blame modern medicine as ineffective.

The obese are not physically fit. They always feel tired and exhausted. They lose their self-confidence and start being ashamed with the guilt of being accused of lack of control and will power. Then they tend to make a decision of losing weight, which may put them in misery and suffering. There are many reasons for it.

- The obese have large bodies and they need a lot more energy to keep their optimum body temperature.
- Also, carrying a heavy, big body is not a simple task. These people need more muscular effort than normal weight people, to move their bodies.

But, this actually does not mean that fat people need more food to eat.

Physicians say that many obese patients gain weight even when they are on special diets, which provide less energy than their actual needs. Therefore, it is very clear that there is some other mechanism which makes them obese. Among the many theories about this hidden mechanism, the glandular theories became very popular.

# CHAPTER TWO

# Glandular Theories on Obesity

There was a time, where the scientists and physicians thought that this secret mechanism is connected with sexual hormones and the functions of their endocrine glands. Some clinical co-relations supported it and they are;

- Many young patients who are obese showed an under development of their sex organs.
- Men used to develop obesity in their mid-ages
- Women put on mostly after their menopause.

But, when the modern medicine introduced highly active sex hormones to the world, the theories of sex hormones became untrue. The physicians found out that obesity could not be controlled even after administrating these highly active hormones.

Thyroid

Then People tried to reduce weight of obese, by administrating thyroid hormones or thyroid gland and thought by that they could break down the abnormal fats in the body, as the thyroid is responsible for body's energy production. Anyhow, this was unsuccessful and we know why. The body's energy is brought by the normal fat reserve and to reach the abnormal fats without touching structural fats, a person need to starve severely.

Many obese people have a normal thyroid gland. It is very rare we find obese with hype-reactive thyroid gland or the other. Treating any of these diseases would not let us cure obesity and also giving a thyroid gland for a diseased or a normal person is useless and dangerous.

Pituitary

The anterior lobe of the pituitary or the hypophysis is the next gland suspected of carrying out this mysterious mechanism of developing obesity. There were no scientific findings proving such a thing even after many studies, except the one on fat-mobilizing factor which is being released. But, it is too early to say whether it is liked with obesity or not.

Adrenals

As Cushing's Syndrome – a disease which leads to a production of high levels of hormones, showed signs which resemble obesity, many people thought they found the real reason. But, decreasing the adrenal functions didn't have any practical mean and also they didn't find increased activity of adrenal glands in obese patients.

The Diencephalon

This is the part of the brain, which controls all automatic functions of the human body such as breathing, heart rate, digestion, sleep, sex and others. This part of the brain is hugely connected with the other endocrine glands. It is well known that the diencephalon carries the center which regulates the sugar level of the blood. Also during certain studies, it showed that destruction of a certain part of the diencephalon resulted in a huge food crave and weight gain in animals which does not get fat normally.

# CHAPTER THREE

# The Causes of Obesity

Among the many causes said to be the reason why people develop obesity, there are 3 main reasons which play a great role, and they are

## 1.  Inheritance

Some people have congenitally low diencephalic capacity and it will contribute to obesity by reducing the fat banking capacity. The fats which are in the normal storage are then transferred to the abnormal fat store. When this is present, obesity will develop at an early age, even when a person has a normal feeding.

## 2.  Diencephalic disorders

Some people also develop different diencephalic disorders, which may lead to lowering of the diencephalic fat banking capacity.

This is visible when the hypothalamus is overworked as in menopause and castration. At this period the sex hormone levels of the body decreases and the hypothalamus overworks in order to stimulate the non-functioning or non-responsive ovaries, to secrete normal levels of sex hormones. This is actually a big burden. The hypothalamus takes a lot of energy from many other centers such as the fat banks reducing its functioning ability.

This is same in the presence of diabetes, when the sugar level is high. They are converted to fat and stored, rather than handing them over to the sugar-regulating center. But, when the diencephalic fat banking capacity is low, these fats, which are converted from sugar, are then deposited in the abnormal fat stores causing obesity.

### 3.  Exhaustion of the fat bank

The third cause of obesity is the overload of work on the fat bank. It happens when the normal diencephalon is overloaded with excess of food or when the consumption of fuel is less. This situation can be explained by taking many examples;

- When a sportsman rest for weeks on a bed due to a muscle strain or a fracture, they increase their body weight rapidly.
- When a person who has adapted to cold climate comes to a tropical country, they put on as their fuel is not used to heat the body up as earlier.
- And also when an active worker start working in one place with the computer, we see again the same issue rising up.
- Another good example is when a person who eats unrefined food starts eating refined food, they start getting fat. This is because the unrefined foods digest and assimilate in the intestines slowly than the refined food. When refined foods are consumed suddenly, there

is a diencephalic overload which will result in obesity.

Other than the above main three causes, there are some others which are of a great concern;

## 4.  Psychological aspects

The diencephalon, which is situated in the brain controlling metabolic functions, is also responsible of human emotions and instincts. Just as it can consume energy from different centers, during a psychological stress, the energy can be switched from one center to the other. That is why lonely, unhappy people are prone to have obesity than the happy ones. Correcting the psychological aspects of these people will correct their body weight, in this situation.

## 5.  Hunger misunderstood as compulsive eating

Most obese patients do not suffer from any eating disorders. Yet, the society has been really unfair in blaming them. It is a genuine hunger which is stimulated by the alcohol, nicotine, sweets and pastries make them eat more.

There are patients who suffer from compulsive eating as well. But, they are rare. This occurs mostly in girls of late teenage and early twenties. This eating disorder makes people crave for food and forces them to eat in large amount and fill their stomachs regardless of hunger. The way they consume food during an attack of compulsive eating, is really fearsome to see.

Compulsive eating is a result of strong sex stimulation most of the time. The strong pressure in the center of sex is transferred to another center which controls the human food consumption. Thereby, this unresolved sex stimulation comes out as an episode of sudden large amount of food consumption. This can be cured by uninhibited sex. But, using uninhibited sex as a therapeutic procedure has its own pros and cons.

A person cannot be recognized of having compulsive eating until they have started getting treatments. The people who suffer from this eating disorder show at least one attack during the treatment.

### 6.  Refusing to lose weight

Even though many think obesity as a minus for their lives, there are some who think it as something dear. Some think it makes them safe, accepted only for their talents and they also think that it makes them stay out of troubles. Also, there are some people who are deeply attached with the obesity they have and think losing weight is like to lose a precious thing in their lives.

Anyhow, these patients need psychotherapy in order to help them see the bigger picture.

### 7.  Just about to get it...

Sometimes when a slim figured woman complaints the doctor that she is getting fat, the doctor might ignore it most of the time. Even sometimes a doctor might write something down for her; while another one check her Body Mass Index (BMI) in order to prove that she is not obese. But, very rarely a doctor notices that she has signs of potential obesity and is just about to be obese. These doubts of a patient about putting on, are right most of the time.

# CHAPTER FOUR

# Signs and symptoms

There are many signs and symptoms of obesity, just like in many other medical diseases. They can be divided into 2 types.

1. Which develop before puberty – it has a strong genetic influence
2. Which manifest at the onset of the disorder

Among many signs and symptoms, there are some, which we actually see in many people and do not think that they predict a future obesity. There are some unbelievable signs which will predict your future body weight;

- Large size of the upper two front teeth.
- Dimples just above the buttocks on the sacral bones.
- Sharp outward angle between the arm and forearm when the arms are outstretched with palms upwards.
- The knock knees.

Other than these signs, there are also some, which are visible at the beginning of the process of being obese and they are;

- Appearances of a small fat pad just below the nape of the neck, which is known as Duchess' hump.
- The accumulation of fat in front of the armpits. The small triangular pads of fats.
- Skin striations which are purple when they are new, and white, later. They appear in hips, breasts and shoulders.
- Fat pads on the inside of the knees.
- Fold of skin over the pubic area.
- A free round skin fold in both sides of chest.
- In men, the development of breasts.

These symptoms can be present in any numbers, and even in people who have a normal body weight and are on a strict diet.

The other clinical symptoms which appear are.

- Frequent headaches
- Insomnia
- Rheumatic pains
- Lethargy
- Frequent hunger
- Irresistible yearning for sweets and starches
- Alcohol consumption
- Constipations
- Menstrual disorders

In a case of slim woman or a man complaining frequently about getting fat, it is important to check for sufficient evidence as above. The presences of few of them are enough to prove that the patient is right. The next thing is that many doctors try to judge obesity through the patient's body appearances when they are with clothes. But, truly, it can be only detected when a person is totally nude.

Dr. Simeons has once consulted a patient who was thin showing ribs, collar bones and dry skin over the cheekbones and jumped into the conclusion that she has cancer. But for his surprise, she showed her hips in which the fat has been accumulated severely. This has been a case of severe dieting. It has taken several weeks for her to recover and look normal. The weight was the same, but the fats were equally distributed in the body, making her look fresh and lively.

Even though a person is underweight, he/she might be suffering from a disorder causing obesity. Likewise, an overweight person may not be having obesity and may show ups and downs of the weight as he/she increases and decreases the intake of calories.

# CHAPTER FIVE

# Treating Obesity

Treating obesity has always been a controversial topic. As obesity is due to a deficiency of the diencephalic center, the only treatment option, a person has is to correct it.

It is not possible to cure inherited genes, and the only way to treat, has been by medications. But, among the many medications acting on the diencephalic brain, none of them showed to have an effect on the fat-center. Even the appetite reducing drugs called as "amphetamines" did not show any positive results.

The "Fat boys"

These boys are called as "fat boys", as they suffer from extreme obesity and sexual underdevelopment. But, their anterior pituitary lobe seemed to be normal, unlike in the boys who suffer from "Froehlich's disease" in which, there is an abnormal growth of the anterior pituitary lobe.

These boys have long, slender hands and breasts, large hips, buttocks and thighs with striations. They also have knock knees and underdeveloped genitals or un-descended testicles.

These boys were treated with HCG (Human Chorionic Gonadotrophin) hormone, which are produced by the placenta of a pregnant woman. The name of this hormone means that chronic – produced by the placenta and gonadotrophin - directed to the functions of the sex glands.

During the study Dr. Simeons did in India, he has found 3 interesting things.

1. Fresh pregnancy urine given by retention enema showed the same results as giving the pure substances.
2. Small daily doses were more effective than larger weekly doses.
3. The patients lost their voracious appetite when they were given small daily doses.

The most important thing, among these three findings was that these patients did not lose or gained weight. But, of course, they changed the body shape - their hip circumference reduced.

The Abnormal Fats on the Move

Dr. Simeons explains the change of the body shape, as the movement of fats from the abnormal fat stores. He says that these fats are being used as fuel under this condition. That is why a 'fat boy' who were administered with daily small doses of HCG, possibly stayed without a feeling of hunger, even when he was on a restricted diet.

It is surely the abnormal fats that circulated and used, because the patients had a good subcutaneous fat layer making them look fresh and lively. There seemed to be no side effects of HCG administration and also showed very good results.

This was the point which brought up the idea of using HCG as a treatment for all forms of obesity. After many cases, a serious doubt arose whether this was the 'dream drug' for obesity. Moreover, the patients who were administered daily small doses of HCG started saying that 250 calorie meal which they were allowed to take, was also too much for the day as they had a feeling of fullness throughout the day.

Pregnancy and Obesity

Even though many people seem to get fat during pregnancy, just because they consume double the amount of food thinking that they have to 'feed two mouths' and they need to gain strength to deliver the baby, the truth is that the pregnancy is the one and only physiological time period in which an obese person can lose weight.

Yes, a woman can get fat during pregnancy, but not obese. The placenta secretes large amounts of HCG during pregnancy and this hormone, as stated before, put the abnormal fats on the move. Actually, this hormone helps wasting all those accumulated abnormal fats and they are used in the body as fuel.

A growing fetus needs nutrition all the time and to supply this continuous nutrition, it is important that mother's blood carries nutrition every second. How is it possible with meals and several hours of intervals without food? That is actually one of the functions of HCG. This hormone maintains the nutrition or fuel levels in the mother's blood constantly. That is why the baby does not starve at any point. This continuous fuel levels are maintained by breaking down the abnormal fat stores, which were locked earlier.

Hence, it is proved that HCG increased the diencephalic fat-banking capacity – actually, it is better to mention the capacity as 'unlimited'. But, when HCG is used as a treatment for obesity, there is no fetus to consume all those broken down fuel. That is why, it is necessary to have a strict diet restriction throughout the period of treatment.

# CHAPTER SIX

# The Gonadotrophins

Human Chorionic Gonadotrophin (HCG)

This hormone can only be found in a woman during pregnancy. But, in a man's lifetime, it is never found. This hormone is produced in large quantities in the placenta and a huge amount is also excreted with urine. There are chorionic gonadotrophins produced by animals, but, they are easily degraded than the human gonadotrophins. Hence, the animal gonadotrophins are very much less suitable for the treatment of obesity.

The name of the HCG brings a misleading idea about this hormone. As according to the name 'gonadotrophin', it is meant that this hormone stimulates the sex glands. But, many years ago, it was found that HCG has an ability of only rendering infantile sex glands into mature sex glands. HCG, in any amount, cannot stimulate a normal sex gland.

HCG was discovered more than half a century ago. At that time the only thing we knew it did, was helping the doctors to detect a pregnancy by excreting themselves in urine. But, as the science developed, there are many researches carried out to find out many other functions of this precious hormone.

Even though a pregnant woman produces millions of IU of HCG per day, 25 IU of HCG is sufficient to lose a pound per day. Isn't it extraordinarily potential? Yes, this exaggerated flooding of HCG in the body is the mere reason why the pregnancy is carried out until the end of the normal term, while protecting the mother and the fetus.

The Real Gonadotrophins

There are 02 hormones, named as FSH and LH which are secreted by the anterior pituitary gland. They are the real gonadotrophins as they directly act on the ovaries. But, the anterior pituitary is controlled by the diencephalon and administration of HCG increases the diencephalic capacity. In sexual deficiencies, administration of HCG will fulfill all the demands of curing obesity as well as correction of sexual deficiencies.

As the action of HCG is on the diencephalon, it is better if we can call it chronic diencephalotropin.

HCG – Not a Sex Hormone

When people hear the word 'hormone', they jump into the conclusion that it has something to do with the 'sex-phere'. But, actually every hormone does not have anything to do with the 'sex-phere' of a human being. Hormones like insulin, thyroid and cortisol, has their own set of functions to carry out.

Therefore, it is important to know that administration of HCG;

1. Has a same effect on men, women, children and elder people.
2. Can only improve any pre-existing sexual deficiencies after the puberty and never stimulate sexual functions beyond normal.
3. Can facilitate conception and regulate menstruation via an indirect mechanism.
4. Will never feminize a man or virilize a woman.

5.  Does not make men grow breasts nor it interfere with the virilization.
6.  Never makes a woman grow beard or develop gruff voice.


Therefore, Dr, Simeons believes that using HCG as a treatment for obesity has no negative effect on the sex-phere of a human being.

The HCG Injection

HCG comes as a dry powder which is extracted from the urine of a pregnant woman. This is less stable once it is dissolved in a solution.

The injection is completely painless and does not result in any tissue reaction. Very fine needles are used to inject this hormone and it is injected deeply into the intra-gluteal muscles in the upper quadrant of the buttocks.

HCG Treatment vs. Other Conditions

**Fibroids**

Normally fibroids do not get affected during treatment except the very large, palpable uterine myomas. This is due to fats, breaking down. Hence, it is better to get large myomas operated before the treatment starts.

**Gall Stones**

Small stones with previous symptoms of colic pains may get frequent colic pains during the treatment. This is due to the absence of fats in the diet and we know that fat is needed for the emptying of the gall bladder. Surgical removal of the gall bladder should be done before the beginning of the HCG treatment.

**Teeth & Vitamins**

Patients with poor teeth sometimes may get troubled during the treatment as just as it happens in a pregnancy. Then the patient is given calcium and vitamin D.

Vitamin C is also permitted to take, which is given in large doses during any appearances of common cold. There is no objection of giving antibiotics in case of presence of an infected tooth.

### Alcohol

The obese heavy drinkers do really well during the treatment. They do not feel to take alcohol like before, while the people who even try to take as a habit can drink only a very small amount. But, the previous urge to drink alcohol returns back when the HCG treatment is ended.

### Cardiovascular Diseases

Actually, this is not a contraindication for the HCG+diet treatment. Patients who suffer from these diseases show an improvement during the treatment, surprisingly.

### Tuberculosis

Patients who suffer from an inactive form of Tuberculosis can be safely treated and there are no immediate relapses recorded in these patients after stopping the treatment

### Painful Heel

The heel pain is a very common complaint of the patients who desperately try to lose weight by dieting and exercising. But, neither the orthopedic surgeons nor the rheumatologists can help this condition.

The most amazing thing is that the HCG+diet treatment can actually heal this heel pain. It is found that this heel pain occurs due to the reduction of fat pad of the heel, because, in these patients the heel shows a softening and the bone is also easily palpated.

When HCG+diet treatment is carried out, the patients say that this heel pain has vanished away completely after about the 15th day of treatment and did not recur even after the end of the treatment.

This draws more attention towards the possible functions of the HCG hormone, as this reduction of heel pain proves that HCG does not only break down bad fats, but also restore the normal fats in the correct locations.

• 21 •

# CHAPTER SEVEN

# Obesity Complicating Disorders

There are many diseases in which the obesity is precipitated as a result. The most important of them are diabetes, gout, rheumatism and arthritis, high blood pressure and hardening of the arteries, coronary disease and cerebral hemorrhages.

Even though these disorders are different to each other, there are two things in common and they are;

1. New researches believe that all these diseases have something to do with the regulation of the diencephalic functions.
2. They do not improve or occur during pregnancy

Even if these disorders are present and If HCG and diet can bring about those diencephalic changes, in the obese, which are characteristic of pregnancy, one would expect to see an improvement in all these conditions comparable to that seen in real pregnancy. The administration of HCG does in fact do this in a remarkable way.

Diabetes

In a case of obesity together with long term, stable diabetes, it is possible to stop all anti-diabetic medications after the first few days of HCG administration. Also, it is possible to achieve normal blood sugar levels in about 2-3 weeks. But, this can be observed in brittle-type diabetes where the sugar levels change frequently in large amounts, as in these cases, the pancreas is not able to produce sufficient amounts of insulin, even under the influence of diencephalic stimulation.

Therefore, the patients with the stable-type of diabetes show better results than the patients with the brittle-type during the treatment.

Rheumatism

All rheumatic pains, together with bony lesions vanish away during the time of treatment, without the need of cortisone or salicylates. But, these symptoms return back, once the HCG administration is stopped. This is the same phenomenon in pregnancy.

Moreover, the HCG administration stimulates the ACTH secretion in an indirect manner and regenerates the adrenal cortex, which suffers due to chronically administered cortisone, as a treatment for rheumatism.

Cholesterol

When talking about the cholesterol levels, the HCG has a positive effect on this matter as well.

There are two types of cholesterols and they are free cholesterols and esterified cholesterols. The latter is the culprit of many coronary, arterial and heart diseases. But, for our great surprise, the clinical administration of HCG showed an elevation of free cholesterols and a reduction of esterified cholesterols. It also shows this change greatly only if the person had abnormal levels. In case of normal levels of free and esterified cholesterol, the change of the levels of each type was not significant.

Gout

The same phenomenon is found in gout as well.

Normally, these patients get an acute, severe attack on the first few days of the treatment and they remain pain free. Some obese patients used to stay free of pain even after they gain their normal body weight. The diencephalic mechanism of gout is unknown. The doctors think it is possibly due to an emotional factor.

These patients are given 2 tablets of ZYLORIC in order to prevent the severe acute attacks of pain during the first few days of HCG administration.

Blood Pressure

The blood pressure drops rapidly during the treatment regardless whether the patient has normal or abnormally high blood pressure. This happens normally during pregnancy as well. Therefore, it is important to reduce the dose or stop the intake of blood pressure reducing drugs, during this treatment. After the HCG administration is stopped, the dropped blood pressure will come back to the previous levels that the patient had earlier.

But the former high levels are rarely reached, and according to Dr, Simeons' impression such relapses respond better to orthodox drugs such as Reserpine than before treatment.

Peptic Ulcers

The patients show an improvement in spite of the diet they have. This is same as what we observe during pregnancy.

Psoriasis, Fingernails, Hair, Varicose Ulcers

All these conditions improve with the administration of HCG. Psoriasis improves, brittle nails cure, hair fall is reduced and the varicose ulcers are healed.

Hence, we have since treated non obese patients suffering from varicose ulcers with daily injections of HCG on a normal diet with equally good results.

The "Pregnant" Male

When a male patient hears that he is about to get pregnancy hormones and is to be put into a condition which in some respects resembles pregnancy, he is usually shocked and horrified. The physician must therefore carefully explain that this does not mean that he will be feminized and that HCG in no way interferes with his sex. It is important that he understands, the use of this pregnancy phenomenon is used to treat the diencephalic disorder, which is responsible for obesity.

# CHAPTER EIGHT

# The Technique

Warnings

- Do not do the treatment by yourself. It is important that you are observed by a good physician during the treatment, as only a doctor can deal with the interrupting symptoms which may come along during the treatment.
- If you try reducing weight by eating less and taking a few 'shots' it could lead you to a disappointing end or may also put you in serious trouble.
- By treating obesity with the HCG and diet method, perhaps we are handing the most complex organ in the body. So whatever happens in one part could be effected to other parts of the body.
- The doses of administration should be calculated carefully, as high doses can evoke counter-regulations.

History taking

On the very first day of the patient presents for the treatment, it is important to take a detailed general history and note the time when the first signs of overweight were observed. Then it is the time to find the highest weight that the patient had in his life excluding pregnancy.

As a next step, we question the patient and get answers in a simple way, such as "Yes" or "No"

Furthermore, Patient will be asked about medications they were taking for a long period, as some medication and hormones, which are administered for a long time can affect a person's body weight.

The degree of overweight is calculated by using a special table and in women large and heavy breasts are also considered during the calculations.

The duration of Treatment

Patients, who need to lose 7 Kg or less, require 26 days treatment with 23 daily injections. After the last injection next 3 days patient should continue the 500-calorie diet.

Given that, this is a very important part of the treatment. Since, if the patient starts eating normally, they put on weight alarmingly after the treatment finishes.

However, after the last 3 days this does not happen due to the blood is no longer saturated with food. When a patient has more than 7 Kg to lose, the treatment takes much longer. But maximum can be given in a single course is 40 injections.

Immunity to HCG

The reason for limiting the no of injections for 40 is because some patients may begin to develop signs of HCG immunity after a certain period of time and then it may lead to break down HCG and reduce the levels very rapidly.

Moreover, Patients who need only 23 injections may be injected daily, but for the patients who need about 40 injections, can be given only 6 injections a week and leaving out one day which patient chooses, just because of this reason.

Menstruation

During menstruation no injections are given, but the diet is continued. When the menstruation is over, the patient becomes extremely hungry unless the injections are resumed at once.

It is very surprising to see a patient who has continued diet for a day or two beyond the end of the period without coming for injection and then the next day that all hunger ceased within a few hours after the injection. Then the patient once again becomes content and cheerful.

Further injection courses

The patients, who need to lose more than 15.5Kg, must have a second or even more courses.

The second course can be started after a time break of not less than six weeks. Likewise, when a patient has to go through several repeated courses, the time break should be given accurately and accordingly.

Conditions that must be accepted before treatment

- The patient should visit the clinic daily to be weighed, injected and generally checked.
- The patients may reside in a friend's or a relative's place in Rome throughout the treatment period or if not may stay in the hospital itself. Staying in a hotel or restaurant cannot be relied upon giving an accurate diet with the exact calorie amount.
- The patients are free to visit anywhere in the rest of the day after the clinic visit.
- Between the courses the patient gets no treatment and is free to eat anything he pleases, except starches and sugar during the first 3 weeks.
- The patient will have to follow the prescribed diet during the treatment and after the first three days this will cost him no effort, as he will feel no hunger and may

indeed have difficulty in getting down the 500 Calories which he will be given.

Without accepting any of these conditions the patient and even the doctor will have to face very disappointing results at the end of the treatment. Hence, refusal of any one condition will lead to a refusal of the treatment.

A patient can be considered himself as really cured, only when he returns back to his correct weight. But, for people with severe cases of obesity, feels themselves, even when they lose half of their weight and come to us for more. Actually, there are enthusiastic, happy compliments given by the patients all the time rather than the negative complaints.

Examination

Once the agreement is reached, the patient will be examined by the doctor. Here are the points the doctor will note down;

- The size of the first upper incisor
- The size of the pad of fat on the nape of the neck
- The size of the axilla and on the inside of the knees
- The presence of striation
- The presence of a suprapubic folds
- The presence of a thoracic folds
- The presence of an angulation of elbow and knee joint
- Breast-development in men and women
- Edema of the ankles
- The state of genital development in the male is noted

Then an X-ray is done of the brain, to check for any changes in the pituitary gland. Another –ray of the chest and an ECG is also done. A full blood count, uric acid level and cholesterol level and sugar level of the fasting blood are checked too.

Gain before Loss

Patients, whose general condition and appearance is poor, need to eat well for about a week, regardless how much they will gain weight. It is because a patient cannot tolerate 500 calorie diet, unless they have a well-stocked fat reserve.

During the first 3 injections, a patient can eat any amount of food of any type. The injections, which are given at this time period, are called as 'non-effective" while the other injections, which are administered under the diet of 500 calories, are called as "effective". This is because it takes at least 3 injections to make those abnormal fats to start moving.

Putting patients on a forced diet for about a week before the treatment is really hard with the people who were following strict diet plans. A gain of weight about 4-6 ponds at this time, is not unusual.

Patients with good general conditions, without any diet restrictions start forced feeding on the day of the first injection. Some patients say that they can no longer overeat because their stomach has shrunk after years of restrictions. But, we know that it's not true and we insist that they eat frequently of highly concentrated foods such as milk chocolate, pastries with whipped cream, sugar, fried meats (particularly pork), eggs and bacon, mayonnaise, bread with thick butter and jam, etc.

This gained weight will be lost during the 1st–3rdinjections surprisingly.

Starting treatment

In menstruating women, the treatment will start immediately after the period. Likewise, the end of the course of injections should be made before the next period. Normally the injections are stopped 3 days prior to the expected date of menstruation and a normal diet is resumed with the period.

Alternatively, at least three injections should be given after the period, followed by the usual three days of dieting. This rule need not be observed in such patients who have reached their normal weight before the end of treatment and are already on a higher caloric diet.

The diet

The 500 calorie diet is explained as below;

BREAKFAST:

Tea or coffee in any quantity without sugar. Only one tablespoonful of milk allowed in 24 hours. Saccharin or other sweeteners may be used.

LUNCH:

1) 100 grams of veal, beef, chicken breast, fresh white fish, lobster, crab, or shrimp. All visible fat must be carefully removed before cooking, and the meat must be weighed raw. It must be boiled or grilled without additional fat. Salmon, eel, tuna, herring, dried or pickled fish are not allowed.

DINNER :

The same four choices as lunch

Here are the things that are allowed and not allowed while you are in the HCG+Diet treatment plan

| Allowed | Not-allowed |
| --- | --- |
| Juice of one lemon daily | Oil, butter or dressing |
| Salt, pepper, vinegar, mustard powder, garlic, sweet basil, parsley, thyme, marjoram, etc | not more than four items listed for lunch and dinner may be eaten at one meal |
| Tea, coffee, plain water, or mineral water in any quantity | No medicines or cosmetics other than lipstick, eyebrow pencil and powder may be used without special permission |
| fruit or the breadstick may be eaten between meals | All things not listed are forbidden. |

Things to be noted

- Use a letter-scale for weighing, not a kitchen scale.
- Break the two meals if you need.
- At the beginning patients are advised to check every meal against their diet sheet before starting to eat and not to rely on memory.
- Any attempt to observe this diet without HCG will lead to trouble in two to three days.
- Two small apples weighing as much as one large one nevertheless have a higher caloric value and are therefore not allowed.
- Tangerine is not an orange.
- Chicken breast does not mean the breast of any other fowl.

Making up the calories

The diet throughout the HCG treatment should necessarily contain 500 calories per day and not less or more.

The diet stated above works satisfactory in Italy. But, for other countries such as Asia, Africa and Middle East, there is a need of modification to be done.

The diet for the vegetarians should be revised completely and the poultry should be replaced with vegetarian foods.

**Plan Of A Normal Course**

- 125 I.U. of HCG daily (except during menstruation) until 40 injections have been given.

- Until 3rd injection forced feeding.

- After 3rd injection, 500 Calorie diet to be continued until 72 hours after the last injection.

- For the following 3 weeks, all foods allowed except starch and sugar in any form (careful with very sweet fruit).

- After 3 weeks, very gradually add starch in small quantities, always controlled by morning weighing.

Concluding a course

After the 3[rd]day of dieting, since the last day of the injection, the patients may eat anything they need, except the sugars and starches as a rule.

It is important that they weigh themselves every morning after emptying the bladder and before breakfast.

It takes about 3 weeks after treatment for the weight to be stable. But, it is necessary to keep the sugars and starches away. Eating those kinds of food may put the patients again in a state of weight gain. It is important to be careful to remember these restrictions during first 3 weeks after the last injection. Otherwise, it will surely bring very bad results.

If your weight stays within 2 pounds of the weight noted on the day of the final injection, it is considerable. But any slight increment even from one ounce is absolutely unacceptable. Then the patient may skip lunch and breakfast and drink plenty of water. In the evening may eat an apple or two raw tomatoes with a beef steak.

The first days of treatment

Here are the findings a patient may notice during the treatment;

3rd Injection

- The patient will feel quite different. A feeling of already has started losing weigh
- A feeling of always being full and reduced hunger.
- Passes more urine.

4th Injection - Lose up to 2 pounds.

- May get a slight headache. Taking an aspirin tablet will make it go away.

5th– 6th days of treatment

- Weight continues to drop at the rate of 1 pound per day
- The headaches vanish away.

Fluctuations of weight loss

After the 7th– 8th injections, the daily diet loss rate may be reduced to less than 1 pound per day. A reduced urine output may be noticed.

According to statistics, mostly women show these fluctuations as they are entirely related to water retention and elimination of water, which are more noticeable in women. But, the weight loss is resumed within about 2 days.

Faulty dieting

People may believe that a slight deviation from the diet may show a huge weight gain. But, this is an advantage because if a person is not restricting himself to this diet the doctor will detect the weight gain easily and within 2-3 days, during the daily clinic visits.

Vitamins & Anemia

Some patients are scared that the restricted diet and weight loss may put them in a state of lack of vitamins or blood cells. But, there were no such cases encountered during the years of treatment of many patients. But instead, it is easily understood that all the proteins, vitamins and minerals which are stored in the fatty tissues are used in the body when they are broken down during the treatment.

Pounds to inches

Unlike in the other weight loss methods, in HCG + diet treatment, patients show a reduction of waist, abdomen and hip circumference, which has a direct relationship with the no of kilos reduced. Extraordinarily this rate is about 1 cm per kilogram, in most of the patients and this rate can go higher on the first few days of the treatment.

Interruption of weight loss

There are 04 types of interruptions;

1. As mentioned above, first is the stationary reduction of weight loss is due to water retention.

2.  The second is called as a 'Plateau', in which patients may face during 4-6 days, mostly during the second half of a full course. This is noticed particularly in patients who have been doing well and have shown a 1 pound per injection weight loss rate.

This 'plateau' can be broken by giving an 'apple- day' where the patient may eat only apple to the maximum of 6 during a whole day starting from lunch until the next day lunch. Only these six apples can be eaten and may only plain water when they feel thirsty. The next way is by giving a non- mercurial diuretic for a day

3.  In rare cases an interruption of weight loss may occur during a longer period of time. This occurs only in advanced cases and hardly ever during the first course of treatment. This is visible in patient who were obese for a very long (10 years<) in any period of their lifetime.

4.  Menstruation. It has been the most common.

If a pregnancy occurs during the treatment, the women suddenly cease to lose weight. In any case of suspicion of a pregnancy the injections are immediately stopped and checked for pregnancy – HCG urine test only after 5 days of the last Injection. Checking prior to that may lead to false positive results.

It is possible for a woman to use oral contraceptives to prevent pregnancy during the time of treatment.

The Errors

**Dietary Errors**

**Salt:** There is no need to reduce intake of salt.

**Water:** The water intake is encouraged. It is advised to drink up to 2 liters a day during the treatment. There is nothing to do with the water to amount of water retention in the body.

**Constipations:** If the water intake is reduced there is a chance of developing constipations if the patient has a spastic colon. As laxatives are prohibited during the treatment, it is important to regulate bowel cleaning by drinking enough water.

As a food intake is limited with 500 calorie diet, it is normal to pass stools once in every 3-4days.

It is important to investigate deeply if there are no visible dietary errors found in the general discussion. The patient has to be really helpful and also understand that small dietary errors may occur during the treatment and they may not be noticeable by them sales. Hence, being very detailed to the doctor, when discussing about this matter, will help both the doc patient to correct it.

Deliberate lies are not of any use and are surely visible during daily visits when weight shows a continuous rise this will lead to a disappointment for both the doctor and the patient.

## Cosmetics

If no dietary errors found, the doctor will think about any chance of cosmetics use. It is hard to believe, but is true that some oils, creams and ointments are absorbed by the skin and interfere HCG action as if a person has eaten them. Then treatment is very sensitive to cosmetics and therefore the doctors ask patients to pause their use during the treatment.

## Massage

Massages are never allowed during the treatment, as it disturbs the process HCG in the tissues. According to Dr.

Simeons, massage, thumping, rolling or shivering might do harm in this time period.

**<u>Other reasons of weight gain</u>**

Other than cosmetics and dietary error, there are many other reasons for a weight gain during treatment. As example:

- Chewing gums
- Throat pastels
- Vitamin pills
- Severe sun burns
- Heavy physical activities
- Cough syrups.... Etc.

Even though patients do not notice, these things contain sugars which may interfere with the 500 calorie diet

The Voice

Even though people notice a voice change during a general attempt of weight loss through weight loss diets & other criteria, the HCG + Diet treatment shows no change in voice. Actually the patients say that their voice has been improved.

Appetite reducing drugs

They are hardly ever used, as actually there is no need of them during HCG treatment.

Muscular fatigue

At the end of the full course of treatment, some patients may complain that they feel weak. These complain are mostly done by the patients who do not involve in any kind of daily physical exercises.

Even though people think it's because they are losing weight, the actual mechanism is a little bit different. During HCG administration, the fats stored in, between and around muscles break down, making the muscle length increase than before. Therefore, when a person needs to do some work, the muscles need more effort to make a muscle contraction. This is merely a physiological action and of course not a weakness.

The Two Troubles after the Treatment

1. In the immediate post-treatment period, the patient may at once begin to feel much hungrier and even weak. It might become visible in their faces and in such cases the patients are allowed to have a very slight increase in the diet.

2. Some patients cannot believe that they can eat fairly normally without regaining weight, after the treatment. They disregard the post-treatment diet rule of saying no only to sugars and starches and try more or less to continue the 500-Calorie diet on which they felt so well during treatment and make only minor variations, such as replacing the meat with an egg, cheese, or a glass of milk. To their horror they find that in spite of maintaining or losing weight, their weight has gone up.

Relapses

About 60-70% of patients hold in their final weight permanently. Relapses occur mainly due to the negligence. Here are some common mistakes the patients do;

- Not weighing themselves every morning.
- Not carrying the scale with them when they travel.
- Trying to judge their body shape by the fitting of the clothes.

Menopause increases the risk of a relapse until the menopause is completely established. Also, most of the teenagers who suffer from compulsive eating, show relapse as well.

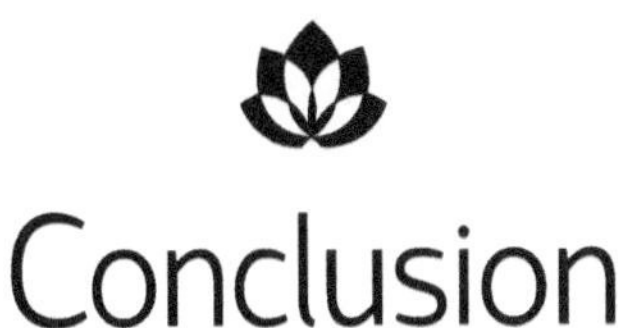

# CHAPTER NINE

# Conclusion

HCG+500 calorie diet is an extraordinary way of eliminating the so called disorder of "obesity", while regaining a healthy and a slim figured body. But, it is not very simple as just getting the injections. It is very important that you maintain discipline and limit yourself to the guidelines.

The procedure is understandable for many, but, the mechanism not. That is why it is important that you talk about this with the doctor before you start treatment. It will allow you to carry out the treatment without any interruptions.

The main advice is that, not to experiment this method by yourself, without a well-practiced physician, as the strict guidelines should be maintained to achieve effective results. In case of a small deviation from the guidelines, may result in serious outcomes.

Obesity is not a disastrous disease like cancer or polio. But, it is serious enough to be treated, as many people today suffer mentally from this. Not only that, but, chronic obesity may result in diabetes, heart diseases and many other metabolic disorders. Hence, curing obesity does not have only a cosmetic value, but also, it makes you healthy and fit.